48 Acne Eliminating Meal Recipes:

The Fast and Natural Path to Fixing Your Acne Problems in 10 Days or Less!

By

Joe Correa CSN

COPYRIGHT

ACKNOWLEDGEMENTS

This book is dedicated to my friends and family that have had mild or serious illnesses so that you may find a solution and make the necessary changes in your life.

48 Acne Eliminating Meal Recipes:

The Fast and Natural Path to Fixing Your Acne Problems in 10 Days or Less!

By

Joe Correa CSN

CONTENTS

Copyright

Acknowledgements

About The Author

Introduction

48 Acne Eliminating Meal Recipes: The Fast and Natural Path to Fixing Your Acne Problems in 10 Days or Less!

Additional Titles from This Author

ABOUT THE AUTHOR

After years of Research, I honestly believe in the positive effects that proper nutrition can have over the body and mind. My knowledge and experience has helped me live healthier throughout the years and which I have shared with family and friends. The more you know about eating and drinking healthier, the sooner you will want to change your life and eating habits.

Nutrition is a key part in the process of being healthy and living longer so get started today. The first step is the most important and the most significant.

INTRODUCTION

48 Acne Eliminating Meal Recipes: The Fast and Natural Path to Fixing Your Acne Problems in 10 Days or Less!

By Joe Correa CSN

We are all familiar with the unpleasantness of acne. It usually comes around in our adolescence and puberty, varying from person to person. Acne can appear almost everywhere on the skin. It usually appears on the face, neck, shoulders, or back. This condition is visually unpleasant. It affects our social life, leaves scars, lowers our confidence, and has a great affect on other everyday situations. Acne can also indicate a serious hormonal imbalance and should be treated professionally.

Acne is often treated with drugs and cosmetic products making it a very profitable industry worldwide. However, these products often don't cure acne the way they should. They temporarily cure the visible part but don't create a significant affect on the cause of this condition.

In order to cure both: hormonal imbalance that causes acne, and to heal your skin once and for all, you will have to dig a little further into what the real problem is.

Studies have shown that the lack of nutrients such as omega 3 fatty acids, carbohydrates, vitamins, and other antioxidants is the real cause.

Healthy, balanced, and well-planned nutritional diets are a universal cure and the true prevention of acne. For example, some foods increase blood sugar, that in turn releases a hormone called insulin. This hormone is respobsible for the increase of oil production in our skin which causes those terrible bumps on the skin. But, by maintaining a healthy diet, you can keep your blood sugar in balance and prevent high oil production on your skin.

I have created this book with acne-specific recipes based on healthy ingredients that are proven antioxidants, high in omega 3 fatty acids, and full of healthy fruits and vegetables in lots of different combinations.

These amazing recipes like Green Soup with fresh asparagus, or sweet Avocado Eggs with cranberries are so amazingly delicious and full of antioxidants that you will be preparing them over and over again. This book offers something for everyone's taste and it's a perfect start up for a new healthy lifestyle without acne.

Let this book be your guide to getting rid of this uncomfortable condition once and for all. Eat healthy and bring back your confidence with healthy and shiny skin!

48 ACNE ELIMINATING MEAL RECIPES: THE FAST AND NATURAL PATH TO FIXING YOUR ACNE PROBLEMS IN 10 DAYS OR LESS!

1. Quinoa Kale Stew

Ingredients:

1 cup of white quinoa

3 cups of fresh kale, chopped

1 cup of green lentils

1 can of tomatoes, diced

1 large onion, chopped

1 cup of fresh celery, chopped

1 medium-sized carrot, sliced

2 garlic cloves, crushed

1 tbsp of vegetable oil

1 tsp of dried oregano, ground

¼ tsp of fresh rosemary, finely chopped

1 tsp of lemon zest, freshly grated

½ tsp of salt

¼ tsp of black pepper, ground

6 cups of water

Preparation:

Preheat the oil in a large nonstick skillet over a medium-low heat. Add carrots, celery, and onion. Pour 2 tbsp of water and cover with a lid. Cook for 10 minutes, or until soften. Add garlic and sprinkle with rosemary and oregano. Stir well to combine.

Add 6 cups of water and canned tomatoes with juice. Add quinoa and green lentils and bring it to a boil. Now, reduce the heat again and simmer for 40 minutes, or until tender.

Add kale and cook for about 10-15 minutes more. Sprinkle with salt, pepper, and lemon zest. Give it a good stir and remove from the heat.

Serve warm.

Nutrition information per serving: Kcal: 290, Protein: 15.1g, Carbs: 48.6g, Fats: 4.5g

2. Pumpkin Puree

Ingredients:

1 cup of pumpkin, peeled and chopped

2 cups of Greek yogurt

½ medium-sized banana, chopped

1 tbsp of flaxseeds

1 tsp of cinnamon

Preparation:

Place pumpkin in a pot of boiling water and cook until soften. Remove from the heat and drain well. Set aside to cool for a while.

Combine pumpkin chops, yogurt, banana, and cinnamon in a food processor and blend until smooth. Transfer to a serving dishes and top with flaxseeds. Refrigerate before using.

Nutrition information per serving: Kcal: 160, Protein: 14.9g, Carbs: 17.7g, Fats: 3.7g

3. Orange Rice Salad

Ingredients:

1 cup of white rice, pre-cooked

1 large orange, peeled and wedged

1 large bell pepper, chopped

2 tbsp of lemon juice

2 tbsp of sour cream

1 tbsp of olive oil

1 tsp of fresh parsley, finely chopped

¼ tsp of salt

4 lettuce leaves

Preparation:

Combine sour cream, lemon juice, oil, parsley, and salt in a mixing bowl. Stir well and set aside.

Place rice in a deep pot. Add 3 cups of water and bring it to a boil. Cook until water evaporates, or until set. Set aside to cool completely.

Now, combine rice and pepper in a large salad bowl. Drizzle with dressing and stir all well.

Place lettuce leaves on serving plates and spoon the mixture into equal portions.

Nutrition information per serving: Kcal: 245, Protein: 4.3g, Carbs: 45.2g, Fats: 5.3g

4. Lemon Salmon

Ingredients:

2 lbs of salmon filets, skinless and boneless

2 medium-sized lemons, sliced

½ cup of lemon juice, freshly squeezed

1 tbsp of olive oil

1 tbsp of rosemary, finely chopped

¼ tsp of black pepper, freshly ground

1 tbsp of sour cream

Preparation:

Combine lemon juice, sour cream, olive oil, rosemary, salt, and pepper in small a mixing bowl. Stir all well and set aside to allow flavors to mingle.

Take a large nonstick baking dish and make a fine layer of lemon slices. Top with filets and drizzle all with marinade.

Put it in the oven and bake for about 13-15 minutes, or until set. Serve with fresh vegetables.

Nutrition information per serving: Kcal: 347, Protein: 44.4g, Carbs: 1.4g, Fats: 18.5g

5. Green Soup

Ingredients:

2 lbs of asparagus, trimmed

1 cup of fresh spinach, finely chopped

5 cups of skim milk

1 cup of chicken broth

2 tbsp of butter

2 tbsp of all-purpose flour

½ tsp of salt

¼ tsp of black pepper, ground

Preparation:

Combine milk and chicken broth in a large saucepan over a medium-high temperature. Add asparagus and spinach and bring it to a boil. Cook for about 10-15 minutes, or until soften. Remove from the heat and transfer asparagus and spinach to a food processor. Reserve the saucepan with milk and broth mixture.

Blend until smooth and set aside.

Melt the butter in a frying pan over a medium-high temperature. Add flour and cook until golden. Pour in the saucepan with milk mixture and stir well. Add blended asparagus and spinach. Stir once again and bring it to a boil. Sprinkle with some salt and pepper to taste.

Serve warm.

Nutrition information per serving: Kcal: 94, Protein: 6.8g, Carbs: 10.9g, Fats: 2.6g

6. Kefir Meat Balls

Ingredients:

1 lb of minced beef

1 large onion, peeled and finely chopped

1 tbsp of fresh rosemary, finely chopped

1 large egg

¼ cup of kefir cream

2 tbsp of all-purpose flour

½ tsp of salt

¼ tsp of black pepper, ground

1 tbsp of vegetable oil

For the topping:

2 cups of kefir

3 garlic cloves, crushed

1 tbsp of fresh rosemary, finely chopped

¼ tsp of salt

Preparation:

Combine the ingredients in a large bowl. Add about two tablespoons of oil in the mixture and shape the meatballs using your hands.

Heat up some oil in a large skillet, over a medium-high temperature. Fry the meatballs for about 10 minutes, or until lightly charred. Remove from the heat and allow it to cool.

Combine two cups of kefir with crushed garlic and fresh rosemary. Top the meatballs with it.

These meatballs are best cold. I suggest you keep them in the refrigerator overnight.

Nutrition information per serving: Kcal: 502, Protein: 31.2g, Carbs: 8.0g, Fats: 38.4g

7. Chia Blueberry Smoothie

Ingredients:

1 cup of almond milk, unsweetened

½ medium-sized banana, sliced

1 cup of frozen blueberries

¼ cup of dates, pitted and chopped

1 tbsp of chia seeds

A few mint leaves

Preparation:

Combine milk, banana, blueberries, and dates in a food processor. Blend until smooth. Add water to adjust a thickness of the mixture and re-blend if needed.

Transfer the mixture to the serving glasses and top with chia seeds and fresh mint leaves.

Nutrition information per serving: Kcal: 281, Protein: 3.1g, Carbs: 29.5g, Fats: 19.7g

8. Eggplant Casserole

Ingredients:

2 large eggplants, diced

2 small onions, diced

1 medium-sized bell pepper, cubed

7 garlic cloves, minced

2 medium-sized tomatoes, diced

1 cup of fresh basil, chopped

½ tsp of salt

¼ tsp of black pepper, freshly ground

Preparation:

Preheat the oven to 375°F.

Place the onions in a large nonstick saucepan over a medium-high temperature. Stir-fry for about 8-10 minutes, or until translucent. Add garlic, pepper, eggplant and about 1-2 tablespoons of water. Reduce the heat to low, cover with a lid and cook for 15 minutes. Add tomatoes and sprinkle with some salt and pepper to taste.

Cook for another 10 minutes, then add basil. Stir well and remove from the heat.

Transfer the mixture to a casserole dish. Put it in the oven and bake for about 25-30 minutes, or until heated trough.

Nutrition information per serving: Kcal: 75, Protein: 3.0g, Carbs: 17.3g, Fats: 0.5g

9. Avocado Spinach Salad

Ingredients:

1 medium-sized avocado, peeled, pitted, and cubed

1 cup of fresh spinach, chopped

1 cup of Iceberg lettuce, chopped

1 medium-sized carrot, grated

1 large egg, hard-boiled, wedged

1 tbsp of lemon juice

1 tbsp of olive oil

½ tsp of salt

½ tsp of black pepper, ground

Preparation:

Mix together lemon juice, oil, salt, and pepper in a mixing bowl. Toss well and set aside.

Combine avocado, spinach, lettuce,carrot, and egg in a large salad bowl. Drizzle with dressing and stir well. Serve immediately.

Nutrition information per serving: Kcal: 324, Protein: 6.0g, Carbs: 13.7g, Fats: 29.3g

10. Banana Dates Parfait

Ingredients:

2 medium-sized bananas, sliced

½ cup of dates, pitted and chopped

8 oz of Greek yogurt

2 tbsp of skim milk

2 tbsp of lemon juice

1 tsp of vanilla extract

1 cup of rolled oats, cooked

Preparation:

Place the rolled oats in a small pot of boiling water. Cook for 3-4 minutes and remove from the heat. Drain and set aside.

Combine yogurt, milk, lemon juice, vanilla extract, and one banana in a food processor. Blend until nicely smooth.

In a serving glass, spoon one layer of the banana mixture, then add few dates and banana slices. Repeat the process with remaining ingredients until done.

Refrigerate 1 hour before serving. Garnish with some extra fruit before serving.

Nutrition information per serving: Kcal: 243, Protein: 9.9g, Carbs: 47.0g, Fats: 2.8g

11. Tuna with Mashed Cauliflower

Ingredients:

5 oz of tuna filets, skinless and boneless

1 large cauliflower head, chopped

2 garlic cloves, minced

1 tbsp of olive oil

¼ cup of cream cheese

1 tbsp of lemon juice, freshly squeezed

½ tsp of sea salt

¼ tsp of black pepper, ground

Preparation:

Place the cauliflower in a pot of boiling water. Cook for about 10-15 minutes, or until fork-tender. Remove from the heat and drain well. Set aside.

Transfer the cauliflower to a food processor. Add cheese and garlic and blend until smooth.

Preheat the oil in a large skillet over a medium-high temperature. Add filets and cook for 5 minutes on each side, or until set. remove from the heat and serve with mashed cauliflower. Drizzle with lemon juice. Enjoy!

Nutrition information per serving: Kcal: 333, Protein: 23.9g, Carbs: 9.1g, Fats: 23.1g

12. Black Beans with Brown Rice

Ingredients:

4 cups of black beans, pre-cooked

3 cups of brown rice, pre-cooked

5 garlic cloves, minced

2 small onions, chopped

1 red bell pepper, diced

1 tsp of cumin, ground

1 small chili pepper, chopped

1 tsp of oregano, ground

½ tsp of salt

¼ tsp of black pepper, ground

Preparation:

Place the rice in a deep pot. add 5 cups of water and cook until water evaporates, or until set. Set aside to cool.

Combine pepper, onions, chili, and 2 tablespoons of water in a large saucepan over a medium-high temperature. Cook for 10 minutes and then add garlic, oregano, and cumin. Stir well and cook for another 2-3 minutes.

Add the beans and 1 cup of water. Sprinkle with salt and pepper and cook for 10 minutes more. Remove from the heat and let it cool for a while.

Serve with beans and rice with lemon slices and sprinkle with some extra salt and pepper if needed. Enjoy!

Nutrition information per serving: Kcal: 484, Protein: 21.5g, Carbs: 94.7g, Fats: 2.7g

13. Turkey with Avocado and Cucumber

Ingredients:

2 lbs of turkey breasts, skinless and boneless, chopped

1 small avocado, peeled, pitted, diced

1 large cucumber, sliced

2 tbsp of olive oil

1 tbsp of lemon juice

½ tsp of salt

¼ tsp of black pepper, freshly ground

Preparation:

Preheat the oil in a large nonstick saucepan over a medium-high temperature. Add turkey and cook for about 10-15 minutes or until nicely browned. Remove from the heat and set aside.

Combine avocado and cucumber in a medium bowl. Sprinkle with salt, pepper, and rosemary to taste. Toss well and transfer to a serving plate, together with meat. Drizzle with lemon juice

and enjoy.

Nutrition information per serving: Kcal: 274, Protein: 26.8g, Carbs: 11.2g, Fats: 13.8g

14. Basil Veggie Pasta

Ingredients:

12 oz of pasta, whole-grain

1 lb of artichokes, halved

1 cup of cherry tomato, halved

1 cup of fresh basil, chopped

½ tsp of salt

¼ tsp of black pepper, ground

2 tbsp of sour cream

1 tbsp of fresh parsley, finely chopped

Preparation:

Cook pasta using package instructions. Drain well and set aside.

Combine artichokes, tomatoes, and basil in a large bowl. Sprinkle with salt and pepper and toss well. Add pasta and stir all together.

Combine sour cream and parsley and stir well. Pour over the pasta and vegetable mixture and give it a good stir. Serve immediately.

Nutrition information per serving: Kcal: 211, Protein: 9.2g, Carbs: 39.7g, Fats: 2.3g

15. Avocado Eggs with Cranberries

Ingredients:

2 large eggs, hard-boiled

1 small avocado, pitted, peeled, and chopped

1 cup of cucumber, cut into bite-sized pieces

¼ cup of fresh cranberries

1 medium-sized tomato, diced

1 tbsp of parsley, finely chopped

Preparation:

Combine avocado, cucumber, and tomato in a food processor. Blend until smooth mixture and set aside.

Cut the eggs in wedges and place them on a serving plate. Pour over the previously made mixture. Top with cranberries and serve.

Nutrition information per serving: Kcal: 202, Protein: 6.1g, Carbs: 9.8g, Fats: 16.5g

16. Sweet Potato Beef Stew

Ingredients:

1 large sweet potato, peeled and chopped

1 lb of lean beef, skinless, boneless, chopped

3 cups of vegetable broth

1 small onion, diced

1 large carrot, sliced

2 small zucchinis, peeled and sliced

1 red bell pepper, chopped

1 tsp of dried thyme, ground

2 garlic cloves, minced

1 tbsp of olive oil

½ tsp of salt

¼ tsp of black pepper, ground

Preparation:

Place the potatoes in a pot of boiling water. Cook for 10 minutes, or until slightly soften. Remove from the heat and drain. Set aside.

Preheat the oil in a slow cooker over a medium-high temperature. Add onion and garlic and stir-fry until translucent. Add carrot, zucchinis, bell pepper, and 1 cup of water. Cook until water evaporates.

Now, add all other ingredients and reduce the heat to low. Cover with a lid and cook for 4-5 hours. Adjust the thickness of the stew adding more water.

Serve warm.

Nutrition information per serving: Kcal: 231, Protein: 27.0g, Carbs: 12.3g, Fats: 7.9g

17. Bulgur Tomatoes

Ingredients:

4 large tomatoes, whole

1 cup of fresh leeks, diced

1 small zucchini, diced

1 medium-sized carrot, diced

1 cup of bulgur, pre-cooked

2 cups of vegetable broth

1 cup of fresh basil, finely chopped

¼ cup of lemon juice

¼ tsp of salt

¼ tsp of black pepper, ground

Preparation:

Preheat the oven to 375°F.

Combine bulgur and vegetable broth in a large pot. Bring it to a boil and cook for 10 minutes. Stir occasionally. Remove from the heat and drain. Set aside to cool.

Scoop the tomatoes and reserve the flesh. Set aside.

Combine leeks and garlic in a large nonstick saucepan over a medium-high temperature. Cook for about 5-6 minutes, stirring constantly. Add bulgur, lemon juice, and basil. Sprinkle with salt and pepper and stir all well. Cook for another 3-4 minutes and remove from the heat.

Spoon this mixture into tomatoes, and place them in a large baking dish. Cover and bake for 30 minutes. Serve warm.

Nutrition information per serving: Kcal: 284, Protein: 6.3g, Carbs: 26.9g, Fats: 1.2g

18. Beans and Onions Wraps

Ingredients:

2 cups of kidney beans, pre-cooked, drained and rinsed

1 large bell pepper, finely chopped

¼ cup of fresh parsley, finely chopped

1 small red onion, finely chopped

3 oz of Greek yogurt

1 tbsp of olive oil

1 tbsp of lemon juice

3 lettuce leaves

Preparation:

Place the beans in a large pot over a medium-high temperature. Add 4 cups of water and cook until soften. Remove from the heat. Drain and rinse well.

Mix together yogurt, lemon juice, and olive oil in a mixing bowl. Set aside.

Now, combine cooked beans, pepper, parsley, and onion in a large bowl. Drizzle with dressing and toss well.

Spoon the mixture into lettuce leaves and secure with a lid. Refrigerate for 30 minutes before serving.

Nutrition information per serving: Kcal: 500, Protein: 31.2g, Carbs: 81.9g, Fats: 6.7g

19. Cucumber Tomato Salad

Ingredients:

1 medium-sized cucumber, sliced

1 cup of cherry tomatoes, halved

1 cup of Feta cheese, crumbled

2 tbsp of extra virgin olive oil

1 tbsp of balsamic vinegar

2 tbsp of lemon juice

1 tsp of vegetable seasoning mix

¼ tsp of salt

1 tsp of fresh rosemary, finely chopped

¼ tsp of black pepper, ground

1 tbsp of fresh parsley, finely chopped

Preparation:

Mix together oil, vinegar, lemon juice, vegetable seasoning mix, rosemary, salt, and pepper in a small bowl. Stir well and set aside to allow flavors to meld.

Combine cucumber, cherry tomatoes, and cheese in a large bowl. Drizzle with dressing and toss well to combine. Sprinkle with fresh parsley and serve immediately.

Nutrition information per serving: Kcal: 183, Protein: 6.3g, Carbs: 6.5g, Fats: 15.3g

20. Grilled Tuna with Peppers

Ingredients:

1 lb of tuna filets, skinless and boneless

4 large bell peppers, cut into strips

1 small onion, sliced

3 tbsp of olive oil

1 tbsp of lemon juice

1 tbsp of orange juice

½ tsp of salt

¼ tsp of black pepper, ground

1 tsp of fresh rosemary, finely chopped

2 garlic cloves, minced

Preparation:

Combine lemon juice, orange juice, rosemary, and 2 tablespoons of olive oil in a large marinade bowl. Add filets and refrigerate for 30 minutes to allow flavors to penetrate into the meat.

Preheat the remaining oil in a large nonstick skillet over a medium-high temperature. Add onion and garlic and stir-fry until translucent. Add bell peppers and cook for 10 minutes or until crisp-tender. Remove the peppers and reserve the pan. Add tuna filets and cook for about 4-5 minutes on each side. Remove from the heat and serve with peppers. Drizzle with remaining marinade.

Nutrition information per serving: Kcal: 352, Protein: 31.7g, Carbs: 11.9g, Fats: 20.1g

21. White Bean Soup

Ingredients:

2 cups of white beans, pre-cooked

6 garlic cloves, minced

1 medium-sized onion, diced

2 medium-sized potatoes, peeled and chopped

1 cup of fresh kale, chopped

4 cups of vegetable broth

½ tsp of salt

¼ tsp of black pepper, ground

1 tbsp of sour cream

1 tsp of vegetable oil

Preparation:

Preheat the oil in a deep pot over a medium-high temperature. Add the onion and stir-fry for 5 minutes, or until translucent. Add garlic and about 2 tablespoons of water and continue to cook for another 2 minutes.

Add vegetable broth, kale, beans, and potatoes. Reduce the temperature to low and cover with a lid. Cook for about 45-50 minutes, or until beans soften.

Stir in the sour cream and sprinkle with salt and pepper to taste. Cook for another 5 minutes, stirring constantly.

Nutrition information per serving: Kcal: 246, Protein: 15.7g, Carbs: 42.3g, Fats: 2.1g

22. Green Tropical Smoothie

Ingredients:

2 cups of fresh spinach, roughly chopped

1 cup of pineapple, chopped

1 cup of mango, chopped

1 cup of coconut milk

1 tbsp of Brazil nuts

Preparation:

Place spinach in a pot of boiling water. Cook for 2 minutes and remove from the heat. Set aside to cool.

Now, combine spinach and fruits in a food processor and blend. Add coconut water and few ice cubes and re-blend.

Transfer the mixture to a serving glasses and top with Brazil nuts.

Nutrition information per serving: Kcal: 348, Protein: 5.1g, Carbs: 30.3g, Fats: 26.3g

23. Salmon Mushroom Wraps

Ingredients:

1 lb of salmon, cut into bite-sized pieces

1 lb of button mushrooms, chopped

2 medium-sized bell peppers, chopped

1 cup of frozen corn, thawed

1 small red onion, chopped

2 tbsp of olive oil

1 tbsp of lemon juice

1 tsp of dried rosemary, finely chopped

1 tsp of sea salt

½ tsp of black pepper, ground

6 lettuce leaves

Preparation:

Preheat the oil in a large skillet over a medium-high temperature. Add mushrooms, peppers, and onion. Cook for 10 minutes or until soften, stirring constantly. Add meat and sprinkle with salt and pepper to taste. Cook for 10 minutes more. Add corn, lemon juice, and rosemary. Stir well to combine and cook for another 2-3 minutes. Remove from the heat and let it cool.

Spread lettuce leaves on serving plates. Spoon the mixture and wrap. Secure with a toothpick. You can add 1 tablespoon of tomato sauce or sour cream. This is, however, optional.

Nutrition information per serving: Kcal: 197, Protein: 18.4g, Carbs: 11.7g, Fats: 10.0g

24. Pumpkin Almond Smoothie

Ingredients:

1 cup of pumpkin, peeled and cubed

1 cup of almond milk

¼ cup of dates, pitted and chopped

½ tsp of vanilla extract

¼ tsp of cinnamon, ground

1 tbsp of flaxseeds

Preparation:

Combine all ingredients in a food processor. Blend until smooth and transfer to a serving glasses. Refrigerate for 1 hour before serving.

Nutrition information per serving: Kcal: 227, Protein: 3.2g, Carbs: 11.9g, Fats: 20.0g

25. Grilled Juicy Beef

Ingredients:

4 lbs of beef steaks, boneless

1 cup of tomato sauce

2 small onions, diced

1 cup of fresh celery, diced

1 cup of button mushrooms, chopped

1 cup of water

2 tbsp of all-purpose flour

3 tbsp of olive oil

½ tsp of chili pepper, ground

Preparation:

Preheat the oil in a large skillet over a medium-high temperature. Add the onions and stir-fry until translucent. Add meat and pour the tomato sauce. Reduce the heat to low and cover with a lid. Simmer for 1 hour until soften.

Add mushrooms and celery. Cook for another 20 minutes.

Meanwhile, combine flour, sour cream, water, salt, and pepper in a nonstick pan over a medium-temperature. Stir and cook for 2 minutes constantly until the mixture thickens.

Stir in this mixture into the pan with meat and cook for 5 minutes more. Remove from the heat and serve.

Nutrition information per serving: Kcal: 393, Protein: 56.0g, Carbs: 4.4g, Fats: 15.6g

26. Baked Potatoes with Onions & Peppers

Ingredients:

5 large potatoes, peeled and halved

1 medium-sized onion, sliced

1 cup of red bell peppers, chopped

1 cup of spring onions, chopped

1 garlic clove, minced

½ tsp of cumin, ground

¼ tsp of salt

¼ tsp of Cayenne pepper, ground

2 tbsp of olive oil

Preparation:

Preheat the oven to 375°F.

Grease a large baking sheet with 1 tablespoon of oil. Spread the potatoes and pierce them with a fork. Sprinkle with salt and cayenne pepper and put it in the oven. Bake for 1 hour, or until nicely soften. Remove from the heat and let it cool for a while.

Meanwhile, preheat the remaining oil in a large saucepan over a medium-high temperature. Add onion, spring onions, and garlic. Cook for 5 minutes, or until onions translucent. Now, add 2 tablespoons of water, cumin, and a pinch of salt. Cook for about 3-4 minutes more, stirring constantly. Remove from the heat.

Pour the onion mixture over the potatoes and serve. You can top with a tablespoon of sour cream. However, this is optional.

Nutrition information per serving: Kcal: 164, Protein: 3.6g, Carbs: 31.8g, Fats: 3.1g

27. Strawberry Flaxseeds Smoothie

Ingredients:

1 cup of strawberries, chopped

1 large peach, pitted and chopped

1 cup of skim milk

1 tbsp of flaxseeds

Preparation:

Combine all ingredients in a food processor. Blend until nicely smooth and transfer to a serving glasses. Refrigerate for 1 hour before serving.

Nutrition information per serving: Kcal: 116, Protein: 5.8g, Carbs: 19.5g, Fats: 1.5g

28. Spinach Quinoa Pilaf

Ingredients:

4 cups of baby spinach, chopped

1 lb of button mushrooms, pre-cooked and chopped

2 cups of leeks, diced

2 garlic cloves, minced

2 cups of vegetable broth

1 cup of white quinoa, pre-cooked

½ tsp of salt

¼ tsp of dried thyme, ground

¼ tsp of black pepper, ground

1 tbsp of vegetable oil

Preparation:

Place mushrooms in a large pot and pour enough water to cover. Cook until soften and remove from the heat. Set aside.

Add 2 cups of water to a deep pot and bring it to a boil. Add quinoa and cook for 5 minutes. Remove from the heat and drain. Set aside.

Preheat the oil in a large nonstick saucepan over a medium-high temperature. Add leeks and mushrooms. Cook for about 8-10 minutes, stirring constantly. Stir in garlic and thyme and cook for another minute. Add vegetable broth, quinoa, and spinach. Reduce the heat and cover with a lid.

Cook for about 15-20 minutes. Sprinkle with salt and pepper and give it a good stir. Remove from the heat and serve.

Nutrition information per serving: Kcal: 135, Protein: 7.8g, Carbs: 22.6g, Fats: 2.2g

29. Apple Acorn Squash Soup

Ingredients:

1 large acorn squash, peeled, seeded, and cut into bite-sized pieces

2 large apples, peeled and chopped

1tbsp of curry powder

1 small onion, diced

2 tbsp of apple cider vinegar

3 cups of vegetable broth

¼ tsp of Cayenne pepper

¼ tsp of black pepper, ground

½ tsp of salt

Preparation:

Place the onion in a large nonstick skillet over a medium-high temperature. Stir-fry for 10 minutes, or until translucent. Now, add vegetable broth, acorn squash, vinegar, curry, and 2 tablespoons of water to the pan. Reduce the heat to low and cover with a lid. Cook until acorn squash soften. Remove from the heat and let it cool for a few minutes.

Transfer the mixture to a food processor. Blend until smooth and return to the pot to reheat. Sprinkle with salt and cayenne pepper to taste.

Serve warm.

Nutrition information per serving: Kcal: 96, Protein: 3.5g, Carbs: 20.1g, Fats: 1.1g

30. Mussels with Veggies

Ingredients:

10 oz of shelled mussels

1 small carrot, diced

1 small onion, chopped

1 medium-sized bell pepper, chopped

2 small potatoes, peeled and chopped

1 cup of fresh parsley, finely chopped

2 small tomatoes, diced

2 tbsp of flaxseed oil

½ tsp of salt

¼ tsp of black pepper, ground

Preparation:

Place potatoes in a pot of boiling water and cook for 3 minutes. remove from the heat and set aside.

Preheat the oil in a large nonstick saucepan over a medium-high temperature. Add tomatoes, carrot, pepper, onion, and parsley. Stir well and cook for 10 minutes, or until veggies slightly soften. Stir in mussels and sprinkle with some salt and pepper to taste. Cover with a lid and cook for about 5-7 minutes more, or until set.

Remove from the heat and serve with pasta or rice. This is, however, optional.

Nutrition information per serving: Kcal: 159, Protein: 2.9g, Carbs: 21.3g, Fats: 7.4g

31. Cranberry Orange Cookies

Ingredients:

1 cup of orange juice

2 cups of all-purpose flour

½ cup of almond butter

¼ cup of apple sauce

2 tsp of baking powder

1 tbsp of cornstarch

1 tsp of salt

2 tbsp of flaxseeds

¼ cup of dried cranberries

1 tsp of vanilla extract

Preparation:

Preheat the oven to 375°F.

Combine all dry ingredients in a large bowl. Add applesauce, vanilla extract and orange juice. Blend all using a hand mixer. Set aside.

Place some baking paper on a large baking sheet. Form the balls or bars and spread over a baking sheet. Place it in the oven and bake for 25 minutes, or until golden brown. Remove from the oven and let it cool for a while.

Serve some melted dark chocolate with the cookies. However, this is optional.

Nutrition information per serving: Kcal: 82, Protein: 2.1g, Carbs: 16.0g, Fats: 0.8g

32. Raspberry Omelet

Ingredients:

3 egg whites

3 free-range eggs

½ cup of raspberries

2 tbsp of tartar sauce

2 tbsp of butter

½ tsp of salt

¼ tsp of black pepper, ground

Preparation:

Combine egg whites and tartar sauce in a mixing bowl. Sprinkle with salt and pepper to taste and whisk with a fork. Set aside.

In a separate bowl, combine eggs and raspberries. Mix to combine and set aside.

Melt the butter in a large nonstick frying pan over a medium-high temperature. pour the raspberry egg mixture and cook for 2 minutes. Add egg white mixture and continue to cook for another 3-4 minutes. Flip the omelet and cook for 2 minutes. Remove from the heat and fold with a spatula.

Serve immediately.

Nutrition information per serving: Kcal: 309, Protein: 14.2g, Carbs: 7.7g, Fats: 25.4g

33. Salmon Pepper Boats

Ingredients:

4 medium-sized bell peppers, seeded and halved

1 lb of salmon, cut into bite-sized pieces

2 medium-sized potatoes, mashed

½ cup of corn, kernels removed

½ tsp of dry rosemary, ground

½ tsp of salt

¼ tsp of black pepper, ground

1 tbsp of oil

Preparation:

Preheat the oil in a large nonstick pan over a medium-high temperature. Add salmon chops and cook for about 10 minutes or until golden, stirring constantly.

Place the potatoes in a pot of boiling water. Cook until fork-tender and remove from the heat. Drain well and set aside to cool completely. Place the potatoes in a food processor and add blend until smooth. Transfer the mixture to large bowl and stir in the corn, and some salt and pepper to taste.

Spoon the potato mixture into the pepper halves and top with salmon. Sprinkle with rosemary and serve.

Nutrition information per serving: Kcal: 154, Protein: 12.8g, Carbs: 14.8g, Fats: 5.5g

34. Peanut Butter Banana Smoothie

Ingredients:

1 tbsp of peanut butter

2 medium-sized bananas, chopped

1 cup of skim milk

¼ cup of dates, pitted and chopped

1 tsp of cocoa powder

1 tbsp of dark chocolate, melted

Preparation:

Combine all ingredients in a food processor and blend until nicely smooth. Transfer the mixture to a serving glasses. Top with melted chocolate and refrigerate for 20 minutes before serving.

Nutrition information per serving: Kcal: 193, Protein: 5.6g, Carbs: 36.6g, Fats: 4.1g

35. Orange Black Bean Salad

Ingredients:

5 large oranges, peeled and roughly chopped

4 cups of arugula, finely chopped

1 cup of fennel, trimmed and chopped

2 cups of black beans, pre-cooked

¼ tsp of salt

2 tbsp of olive oil

1 tbsp of balsamic vinegar

¼ tsp of black pepper, ground

¼ tsp of Cayenne pepper, ground

Preparation:

Place the beans in a pot of boiling water. Cook until soften and remove from the heat. Drain well and set aside.

Mix together oil, vinegar, cayenne pepper, salt, and pepper in a small mixing bowl. Toss well and set aside.

Now, combine arugula, fennel, and beans in a large salad bowl. Drizzle with previously made dressing and toss well to coat. Let it stand for 15 minutes before serving to allow flavors to mingle.

Enjoy!

Nutrition information per serving: Kcal: 256, Protein: 12.0g, Carbs: 45.0g, Fats: 4.4g

36. Sea Bass Stew

Ingredients:

4 sea bass filets, skinless and boneless

4 small onions, chopped

2 garlic cloves, minced

1 cup of parsley, finely chopped

4 cherry tomatoes, diced

¼ cup of green olives, pitted and chopped

2 tbsp of olive oil

1 tbsp of balsamic vinegar

1 tsp of lemon zest, freshly grated

1 tsp of chili pepper, ground

Preparation:

Preheat the oil in a large nonstick saucepan over a medium-high temperature. Add onions and stir-fry until translucent. Stir in diced cherry tomatoes and olives. Cook for about 10-15 minutes. Remove from the heat.

Pour half of the tomato mixture in a deep pot. Make a layer of meat and top with remaining tomato mixture. Stir in the vinegar and sprinkle with lemon zest, chilli pepper, and parsley. Reduce the heat and cover with a lid.

Cook for about 20 minutes and remove the lid. Stir the stew couple of times and add extra salt if needed. Cook for 5 minutes and remove from the heat.

Serve warm.

Nutrition information per serving: Kcal: 173, Protein: 17.6g, Carbs: 9.4g, Fats: 7.6g

37. Greek Yogurt Soup

Ingredients:

1 cup of white rice, pre-cooked

1 lb of Greek yogurt

2 oz of butter

1 tsp of chili pepper, ground

½ tsp of salt

Preparation:

Place the rice in a deep pot. Add 2 cups of water and cook for 20 minutes, or until set. Remove from the heat and let it cool.

Combine rice and yogurt in a food processor. Blend until smooth. Transfer to a serving bowl.

Melt the butter in a saucepan and add chili pepper. Drizzle the soup with this mixture. Sprinkle with salt and serve.

Nutrition information per serving: Kcal: 357, Protein: 14.9g, Carbs: 41.7g, Fats: 14.1g

38. Creamy Beef Balls

Ingredients:

1 lb of minced beef

½ cup of fresh parsley, finely chopped

1 small onion, finely chopped

1 tsp of cumin, ground

1 tbsp of olive oil

2 slices of bread

2 tbsp of cream cheese

Preparation:

Soak the bread slices in water for 5 minutes. drain and squeeze the water and transfer it to a large bowl. Add meat, onion, cumin, parsley, salt, and pepper. Mix all squeezing with hands.

Form the ball-shaped pieces with oil-greased hands.

Preheat the oil in a large nonstick frying pan and fry the balls for about 5-7 minutes or until nicely brown. Transfer the balls to a serving plate. Top with cream cheese.

Nutrition information per serving: Kcal: 270, Protein: 35.7g, Carbs: 5.1g, Fats: 11.0g

39. Green Salad with Greek Yogurt Dressing

Ingredients:

3 cups of Romaine lettuce, chopped

1 large apple, cored and chopped

½ cup of spring onions, chopped

1 large bell pepper, chopped

2 tbsp of almonds, roughly chopped

For the dressing:

¼ cup of Greek yogurt

3 tbsp of olive oil

2 tbsp of balsamic vinegar

¼ tsp of salt

¼ tsp of black pepper, ground

Preparation:

Combine all dressing ingredients in a mixing bowl and toss well. Set aside to allow flavor to meld.

In a large salad bowl, mix lettuce, apple, onions, and pepper. Drizzle the salad with dressing and top with almonds. Add extra salt and pepper to taste, if needed.

Nutrition information per serving: Kcal: 157, Protein: 1.5g, Carbs: 12.9g, Fats: 12.3g

40. Orange Carrot Smoothe

Ingredients:

2 large oranges, chopped

1 large carrot, chopped

1 cup of Greek yogurt

½ tsp of fresh ginger, grated

1 tbsp of lemon juice

1 tbsp of chia seeds

1 tsp of cocoa powder

Preparation:

Combine oranges, carrot, lemon juice, ginger and chia seeds in a food processor. Blend until nicely smooth. Now, add yogurt and re-blend for 1 minute. Transfer the mixture to a serving glasses and sprinkle with cocoa. Refrigerate for 30 minutes before serving.

Nutrition information per serving: Kcal: 121, Protein: 8.2g, Carbs: 20.1g, Fats: 1.6g

41. Spicy Turkey with Eggplant Puree

Ingredients:

2 lbs of turkey breasts, skinless and boneless

5 oz of cream cheese

2 tbsp of olive oil

2 tbsp of lemon juice

2 tbsp of green chili pepper, finely chopped

2 garlic clove, minced

1 tsp of fresh rosemary, finely chopped

½ tsp of sea salt

¼ tsp of black pepper, ground

For eggplant puree:

1 large eggplant, peeled and chopped

2 tbsp of butter

1 cup of skim milk

2 tbsp of lemon juice

¼ cup of cream cheese

2 tbsp of all-purpose flour

1 tsp of salt

Preparation:

Place eggplant in a large bowl. Add milk and lemon juice. Coat well and set aside to soak for 15 minutes. Sprinkle with some salt to taste.

Melt the butter in a large skillet over a medium-high temperature. Add flour and cheese. Cook for 1 minute, or until cheese melts. Pour eggplant mixture into the pan and cook until slightly tender. Remove from the heat and let it cool for a while. Transfer the mixture to a food processor and blend until nicely smooth. Set aside.

Combine oil, lemon juice, garlic and chili peppers in a large glass bowl. Place meat and coat well using a spoon. Refrigerate for 1 hour to allow flavors to penetrate into the meat.

Preheat the grill to a medium-high temperature. Grill for about 7-10 minutes on each side until golden brown. Top with cheese and grill until cheese begins to melt. Remove from the grill and serve with eggplant puree.

Nutrition information per serving: Kcal: 239, Protein: 18.6g, Carbs: 10.2g, Fats: 13.8g

42. African Peanut Butter Stew

Ingredients:

½ cup of peanut butter

2 cups of sweet potatoes, peeled and cubed

1 cup of tomatoes, diced

2 small onions, chopped

1 small zucchini, peeled and chopped

2 small bell peppers, chopped

2 cups of tomato juice

2 tbsp of vegetable oil

2 garlic cloves, crushed

2 tbsp of coriander, ground

1 small chili pepper, minced

1 small eggplant, chopped

1 cup of water

½ tsp of salt

Preparation:

Place sweet potatoes in a pot of boiling water. Cook until fork-tender and remove from the heat. Drain and set aside.

Preheat the oil in a large nonstick skillet over a medium-high temperature. Add garlic, onions, coriander, and chili pepper. Cook for about 1-2 minutes, or until onions translucent. Now, add eggplant, tomatoes, and 1 cup of water. Cover with a lid and reduce the heat. Simmer for about 10-15 minutes. Add peppers and zucchini. Cook for another 20 minutes, stirring occasionally. Gradually stir in peanut butter and tomato sauce and add sweet potatoes. Adjust the thickness with adding more water. Cook for 20 minutes, until potatoes are tender.

Nutrition information per serving: Kcal: 174, Protein: 5.2g, Carbs: 20.1g, Fats: 9.5g

43. Ricotta Beets Salad

Ingredients:

1 cup of Ricotta cheese, crumbled

2 cups of beets, trimmed and chopped

3 cups of arugula, trimmed and chopped

½ cup of orange juice, freshly squeezed

2 tbsp of extra-virgin olive oil

½ tsp of Himalayan salt

¼ tsp of red pepper, ground

Preparation:

Place the beets in a pot of boiling water. Cook until fork-tender and remove from the heat. Drain and set aside.

Combine orange juice, oil, salt, and pepper in a large bowl. Mix well and add beets. Coat well with marinade and set aside for 30 minutes.

In a separate bowl, combine cheese and arugula. Top with soaked beets. Sprinkle with some extra salt and pepper to taste and serve.

Nutrition information per serving: Kcal: 207, Protein: 9.2g, Carbs: 16.0g, Fats: 12.2g

44. Chives Omelet

Ingredients:

6 large eggs

1 cup of chives, chopped

½ cup of Feta cheese, crumbled

1 tbsp of butter

½ tsp of salt

¼ tsp of black pepper, ground

Preparation:

Beat the eggs in a medium-sized bowl. Sprinkle with salt and pepper and whisk until fluffy. Add chives and whisk again to combine. Set aside.

Melt butter in a large nonstick pan over a medium-high temperature. pour the egg mixture and spread evenly. Cook for 2 minutes and flip the omelet. Add cheese and cook for about 2-3 minutes more, or until set. Fold the omelet in half and remove from the heat. Serve.

Nutrition information per serving: Kcal: 372, Protein: 25.1g, Carbs: 3.9g, Fats: 28.8g

45. Guacamole Salmon

Ingredients:

2 lbs of salmon filets, skinless and boneless

2 small avocados, pitted and chopped

1 large tomato, chopped

1 small onion, chopped

3 tbsp of fresh coriander, chopped

3 garlic cloves, minced

½ tsp of salt

¼ tsp of black pepper, ground

2 tbsp of olive oil

1 tbsp of rosemary, roughly chopped

2 tbsp of lemon juice

Preparation:

Place salmon filets in a large bowl. Add 1 tablespoon of oil, rosemary, and lemon juice. Coat well and set aside to allow flavors to penetrate into the meat.

Combine avocados, tomato, onion, coriander, garlic, salt, and pepper in a food processor. Blend until pureed. Transfer to a serving plate and set aside.

Preheat the remaining oil in a large nonstick skillet over a medium-high temperature. Add meat and cook for 5 minutes on each side. Remove from the heat and transfer to a serving plate with guacamole. Add extra salt and pepper, if needed. Serve immediately.

Nutrition information per serving: Kcal: 294, Protein: 23.4g, Carbs: 6.8g, Fats: 20.5g

46. Quick Chicken Stew

Ingredients:

1 whole chicken, (about 3 lbs)

10 oz of fresh broccoli, chopped

7 oz cauliflower florets, chopped

1 large onion, finely chopped

1 large potato, peeled and chopped

3 medium-sized carrots, sliced

1 large tomato, peeled and chopped

A handful of yellow wax beans, whole

A handful of fresh parsley, finely chopped

2 tbsp of olive oil

2 tsp of salt

½ tsp of black pepper, ground

1 tbsp of Cayenne pepper, ground

Preparation:

Clean the chicken and generously sprinkle with some salt. Set aside.

Grease the bottom of a pressure pot with olive oil. Add finely chopped onion and stir-fry for 3-4 minutes and then add sliced carrot. Continue to cook for 5 more minutes.

Now add the vegetables, salt, black pepper, Cayenne pepper, and top with chicken. Add one cup of water and close the lid.

Cook for 45 minutes.

Nutrition information per serving: Kcal: 290, Protein: 31.4g, Carbs: 39.6g, Fats: 6.8g

47. Shallot Omelet

Ingredients:

6 large eggs, beaten

4 tbsp of sour cream

1 tbsp of butter

1 cup of shallots, chopped

½ tsp of ginger, ground

½ tsp of salt

¼ tsp of black pepper

Preparation:

Combine eggs, salt, and pepper in a mixing bowl. Beat well with a fork and set aside.

Melt the butter in a large nonstick frying pan over a medium-high temperature. Add shallots and sour cream. Stir in the eggs mixture and cook for 3 minutes. sprinkle with ginger and flip the omelet. Cook for another 3 minutes and fold the omelet. Remove from the heat and serve immediately.

Nutrition information per serving: Kcal: 377, Protein: 21.8g, Carbs: 16.1g, Fats: 25.8g

48. Lemon Cream Salmon

Ingredients:

2 lbs of salmon fillets, skinless and boneless

2 cups of fresh spinach, finely chopped

2 cups of cream cheese

4 tbsp of lemon juice, freshly squeezed

2 garlic cloves, minced

4 tbsp of olive oil

½ tsp of sea salt

1 tbsp of fresh parsley, finely chopped

½ tsp of black pepper, ground

Preparation:

Preheat 2 tablespoons of oil in a large nonstick skillet over a medium-high temperature. Add fillets and cook for 3-4 minutes on each side, or until golden brown. Remove from the heat and set aside.

In a separate skillet, preheat the remaining oil over a medium-high temperature. Add spinach and cook for about 2 minutes until soften. Remove from the heat and set aside.

In a large frying pan, combine cream cheese, lemon juice, garlic, parsley, salt, and black pepper. Heat it up for 2 minutes stirring constantly, but do not boil.

Combine salmon and spinach on a serving plate. Drizzle all with lemon cream and serve.

Nutrition information per serving: Kcal: 557, Protein: 35.6g, Carbs: 3.1g, Fats: 45.8g

ADDITIONAL TITLES FROM THIS AUTHOR

70 Effective Meal Recipes to Prevent and Solve Being Overweight: Burn Fat Fast by Using Proper Dieting and Smart Nutrition

By

Joe Correa CSN

41 Alzheimer's Preventing Meal Recipes: Reduce or Eliminate Your Alzheimer's Condition in 30 Days or Less!

By

Joe Correa CSN

70 Effective Breast Cancer Meal Recipes: Prevent and Fight Breast Cancer with Smart Nutrition and Powerful Foods

By

Joe Correa CSN

www.ingramcontent.com/pod-product-compliance
Lightning Source LLC
Chambersburg PA
CBHW051034030426
42336CB00015B/2871